The Look Out! Book

A CHILD'S GUIDE TO WATER SAFETY

Cindy Blakely and Suzanne Drinkwater • Illustrated by Barbara Klunder

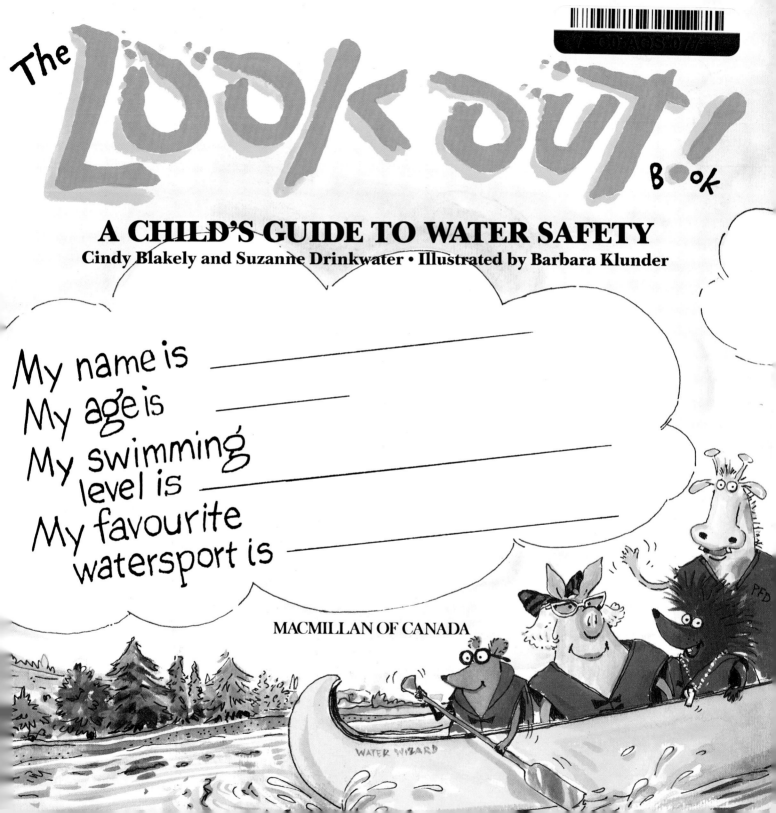

My name is _____

My age is _____

My swimming level is _____

My favourite watersport is _____

MACMILLAN OF CANADA

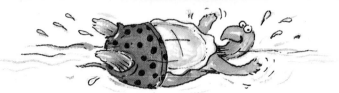

TO A NEW AWARENESS ON THE WATER
Cindy Blakely and Suzanne Drinkwater

FOR THE ISLAND CHILDREN
who are surrounded by water,
with love from Barbara Klunder

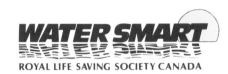

ROYAL LIFE SAVING SOCIETY CANADA

The Royal Life Saving Society Canada (RLSSC) is a national not-for-profit organization dedicated to preventing accidents and saving life in aquatic environments. The Society estimates that over 10,000 rescues are made annually by people with RLSSC training, yet drowning remains the second leading cause of accidental death in Canada to those under 35 years of age.

Water Smart is the theme of the RLSSC public awareness campaign designed to provide basic aquatic safety knowledge and simple personal lifesaving education for use by swimmers and non-swimmers in, on, or near the water.

Cindy Blakely has three children; she is a social worker with special experience in child welfare. *Suzanne McClelland Drinkwater* also has three children; she has been involved in publishing and the world of books for many years. *Barbara Klunder* has one child; she has illustrated many children's books and won numerous illustration awards for her work.

CANADIAN CATALOGUING IN PUBLICATION DATA
Blakely, Cindy, and Drinkwater, Suzanne
        The look out! book: a child's guide to water safety
ISBN 0-7715-9427-5
1.   Aquatic sports – Safety measures – Juvenile literature.
2.   Children's accidents – Prevention – Juvenile literature.
I. Drinkwater, Suzanne. II. Klunder, Barbara. III. Title.
GV770.6.B53 1989   j797′.028′9   C89-095219-1

Media used by Barbara Klunder: watercolour and gouache paints with ink
Editorial design by Nancy Ruth Jackson
Printed in Singapore

Macmillan of Canada
A Division of Canada Publishing Corporation
Toronto, Ontario, Canada

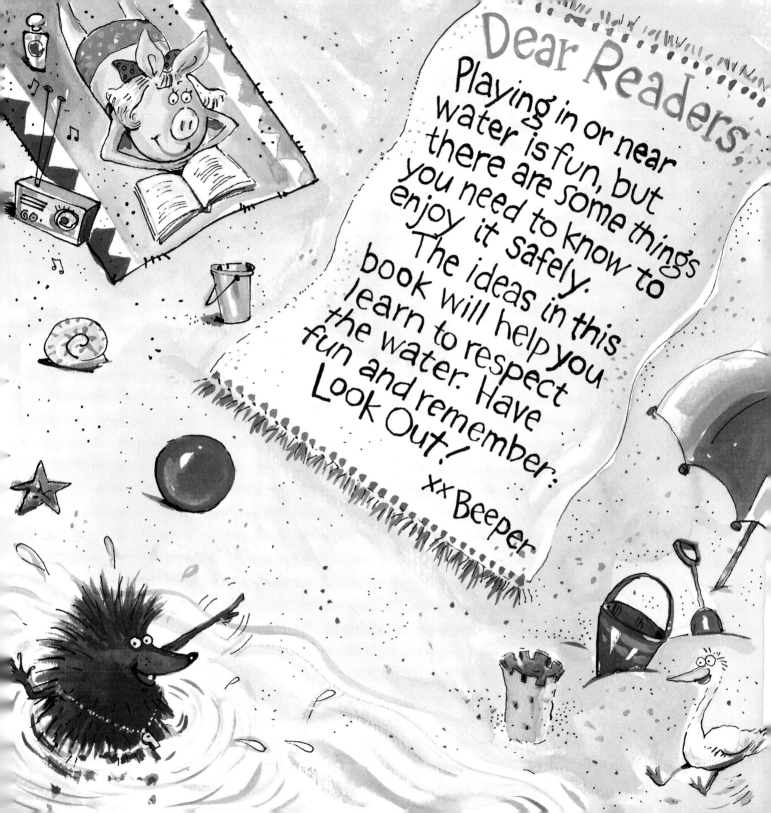

Dear Readers,

Playing in or near water is fun, but there are some things you need to know to enjoy it safely. The ideas in this book will help you learn to respect the water. Have fun and remember,

Look Out!

xx Beeper

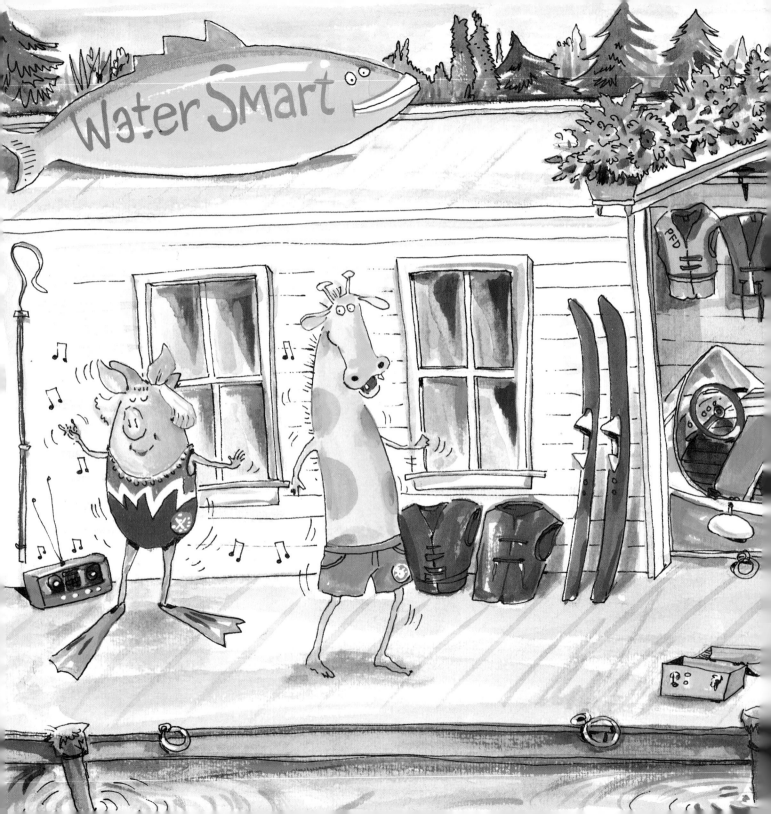

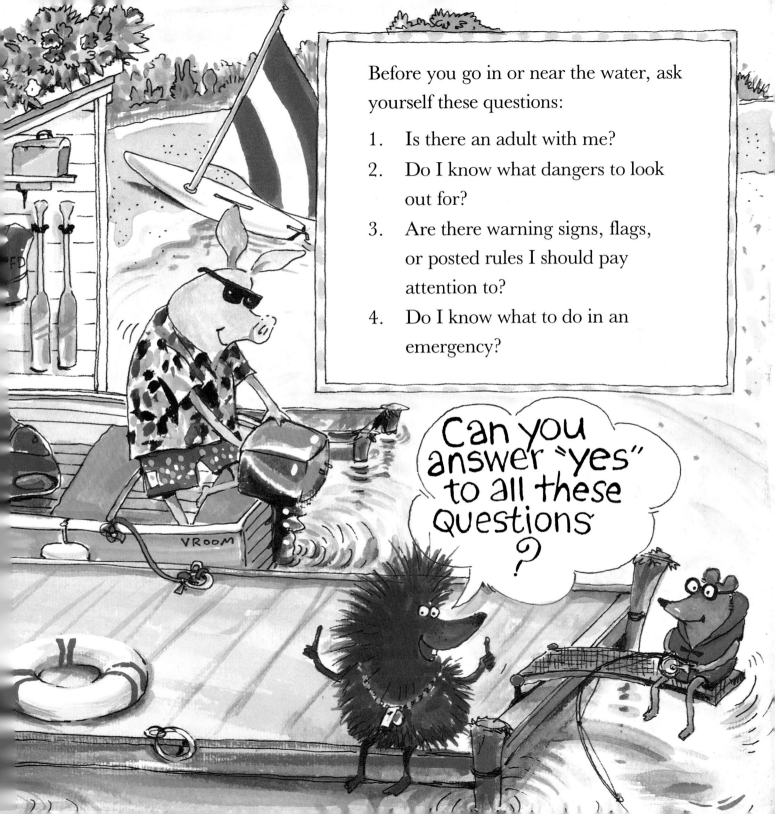

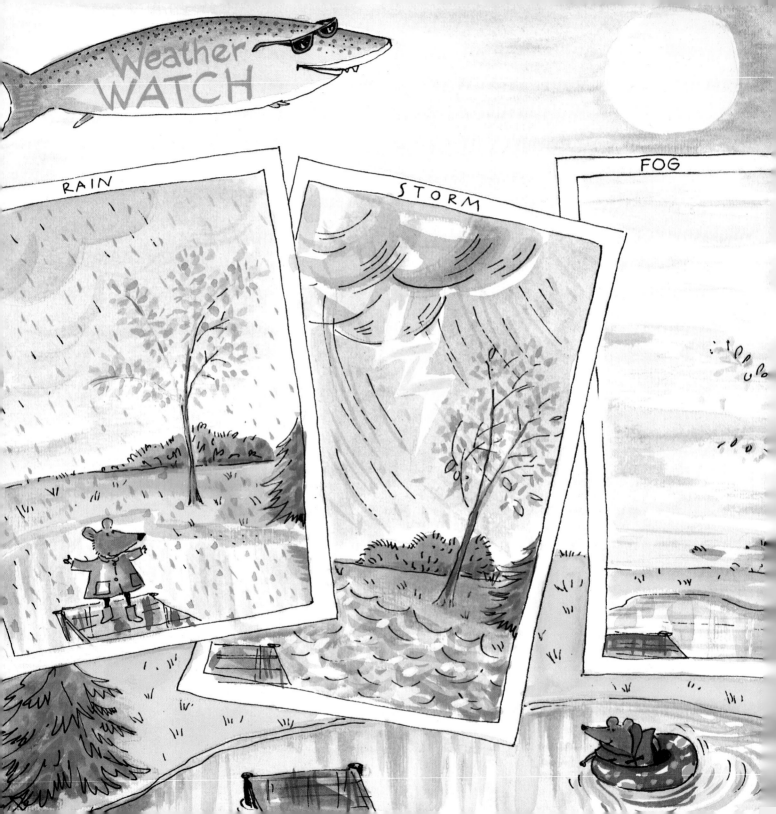

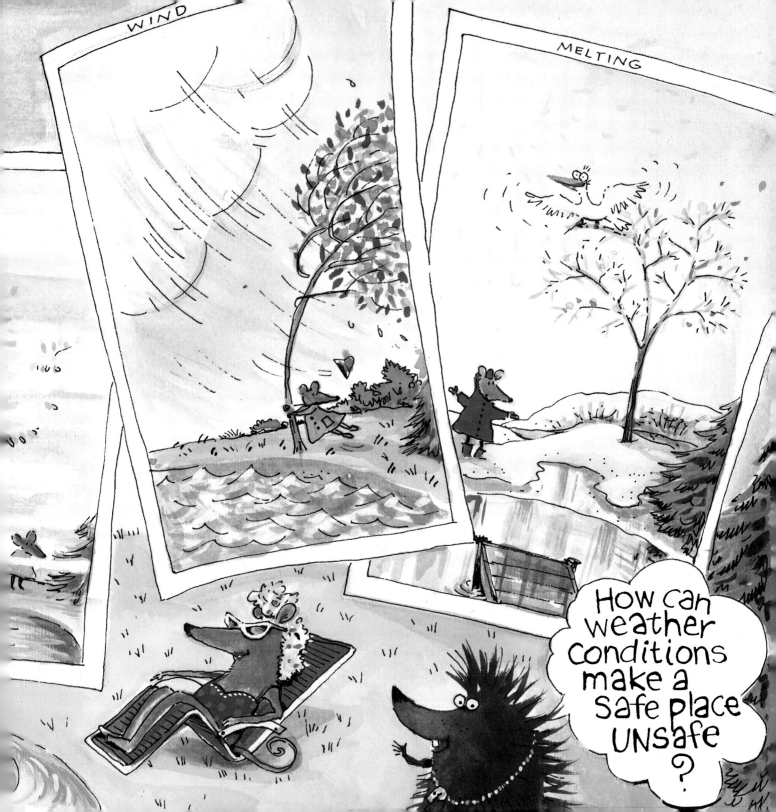

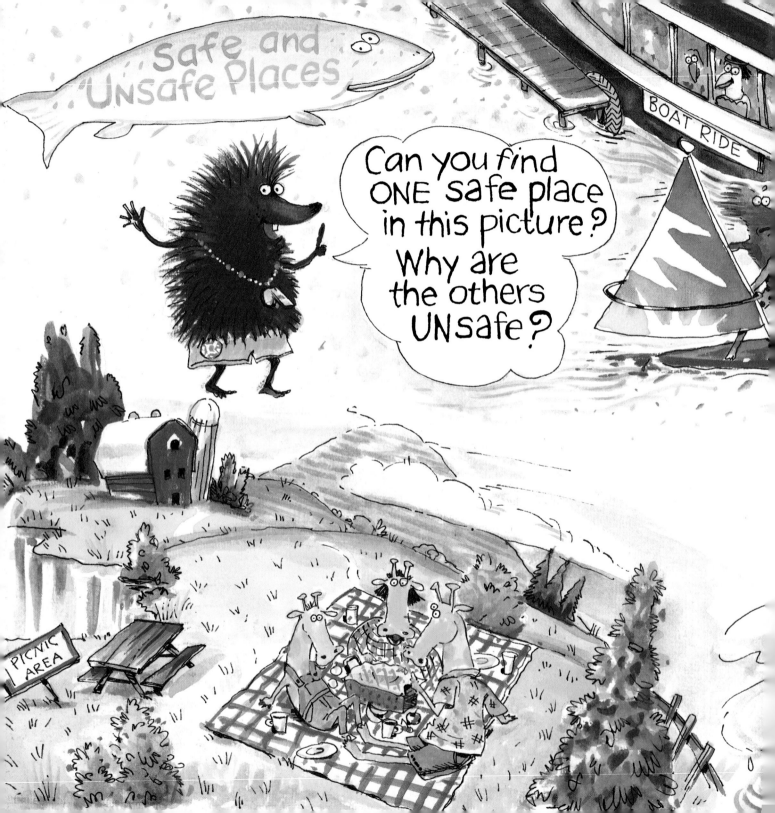

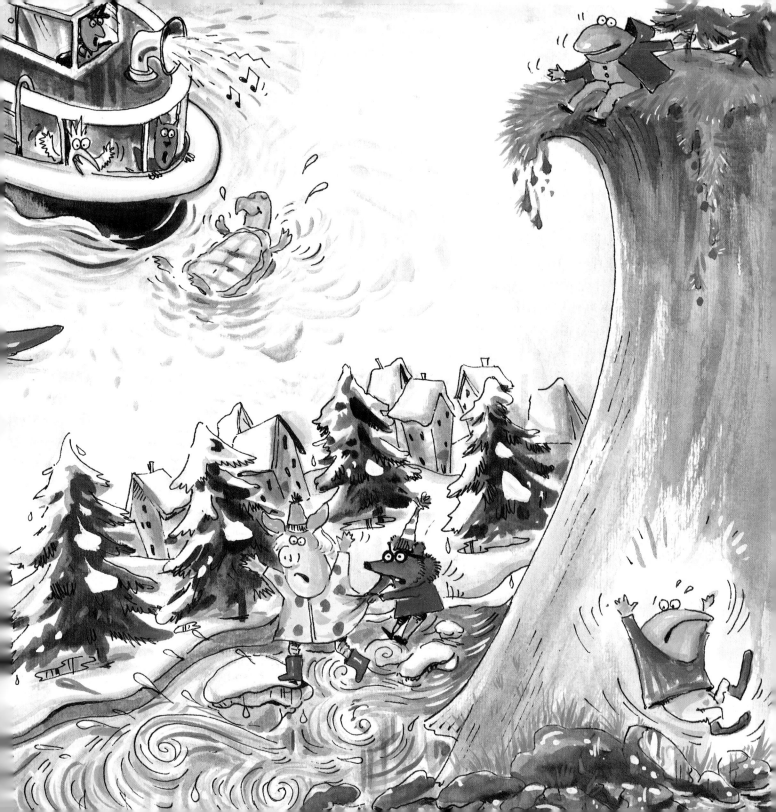

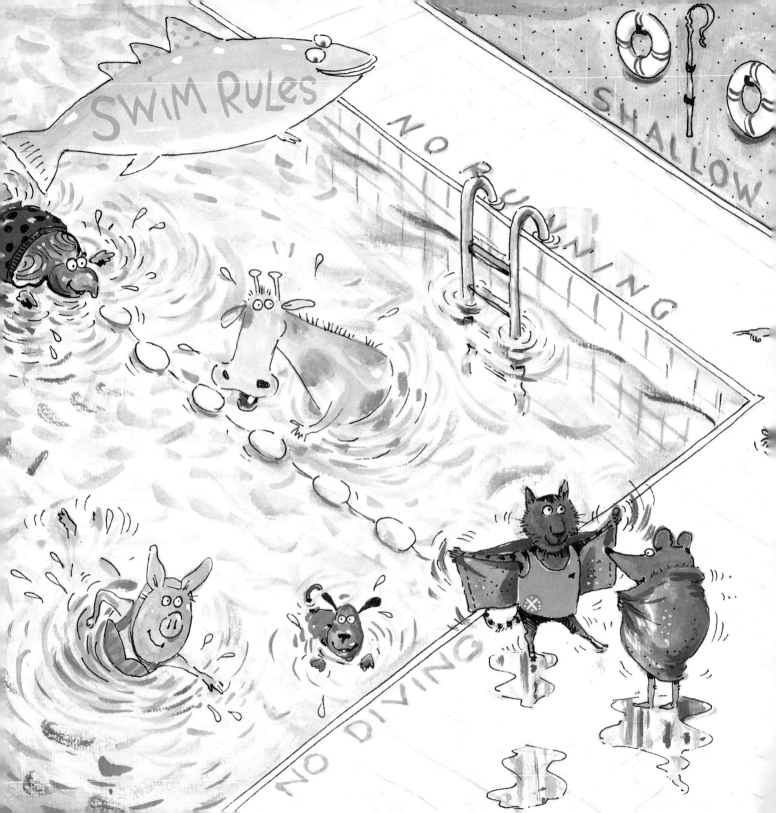

1. Never swim alone. Always go with an adult.
2. Learn how to swim properly. Take swimming lessons.
3. Learn and follow the rules at the pool or the beach.
4. Only swim in a supervised swimming area.
5. Always look before you jump or dive into the water.
6. Never dive into shallow water.
7. Don't run or show off. Never push others into the water or hold them under.
8. Never swim when you are tired or chilled. Don't swim right after eating.

What are the differences between swimming in a pool and swimming in a lake or ocean?

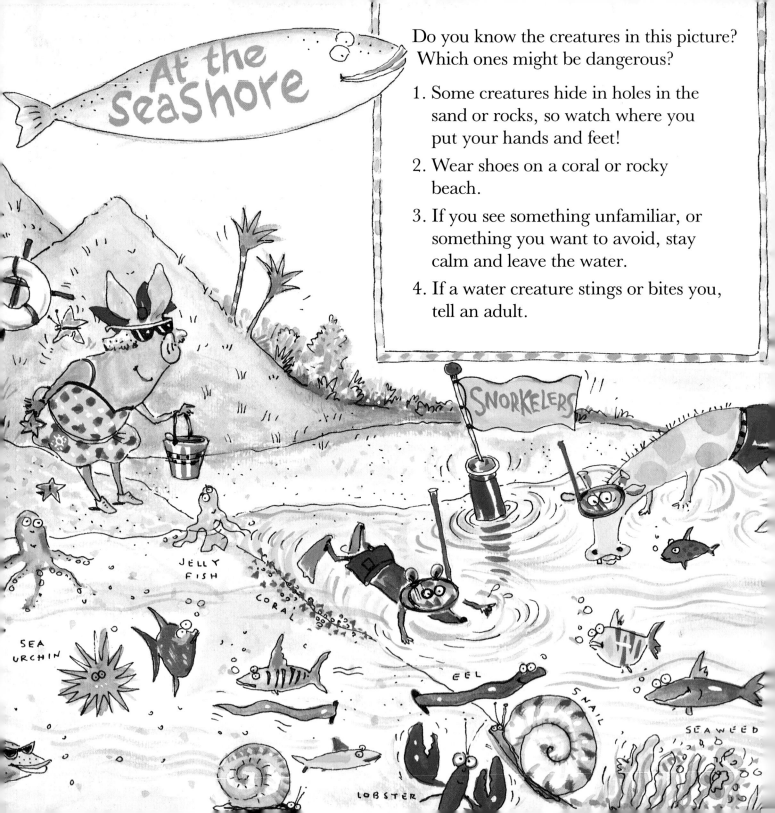

At the Seashore

Do you know the creatures in this picture?
Which ones might be dangerous?

1. Some creatures hide in holes in the sand or rocks, so watch where you put your hands and feet!

2. Wear shoes on a coral or rocky beach.

3. If you see something unfamiliar, or something you want to avoid, stay calm and leave the water.

4. If a water creature stings or bites you, tell an adult.

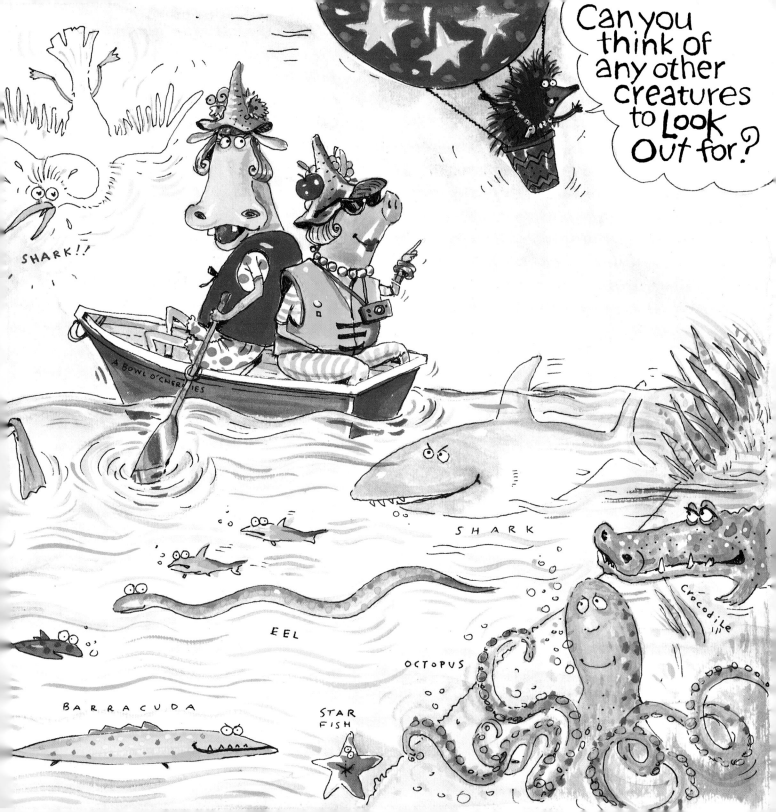

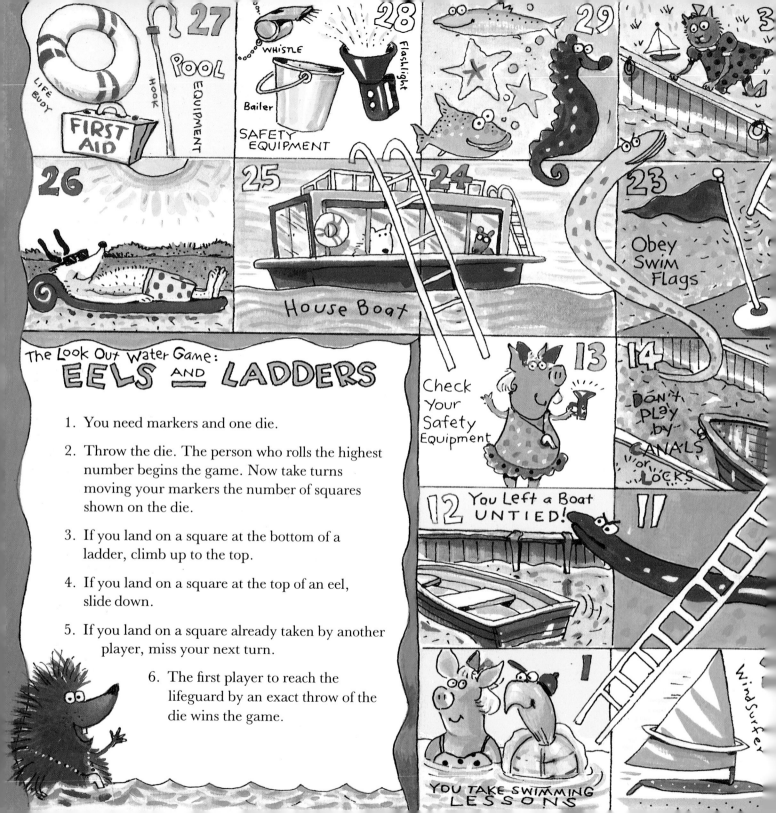

27 POOL EQUIPMENT — LIFE BUOY, HOOK, FIRST AID

28 SAFETY EQUIPMENT — WHISTLE, Bailer, Flashlight

29

23 Obey Swim Flags

26

25 House Boat

24

13 Check Your Safety Equipment

14 DON'T PLAY by CANALS or LOCKS

12 You Left a Boat UNTIED!

11

1 YOU TAKE SWIMMING LESSONS

WindSurfer

The Look Out Water Game: EELS AND LADDERS

1. You need markers and one die.

2. Throw the die. The person who rolls the highest number begins the game. Now take turns moving your markers the number of squares shown on the die.

3. If you land on a square at the bottom of a ladder, climb up to the top.

4. If you land on a square at the top of an eel, slide down.

5. If you land on a square already taken by another player, miss your next turn.

6. The first player to reach the lifeguard by an exact throw of the die wins the game.

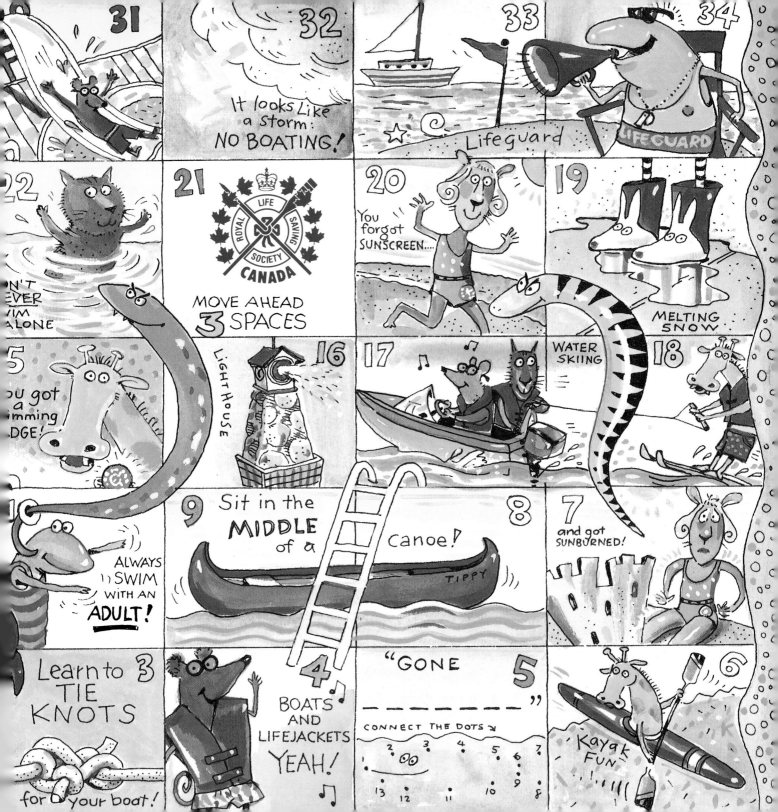

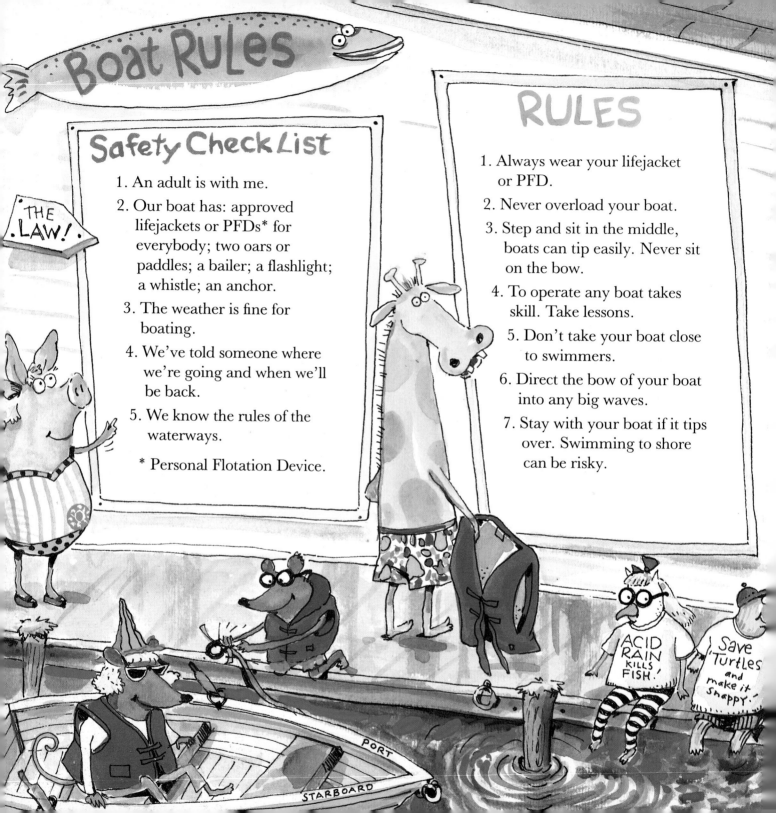

Boat Rules

Safety Check List

1. An adult is with me.
2. Our boat has: approved lifejackets or PFDs* for everybody; two oars or paddles; a bailer; a flashlight; a whistle; an anchor.
3. The weather is fine for boating.
4. We've told someone where we're going and when we'll be back.
5. We know the rules of the waterways.

* Personal Flotation Device.

RULES

1. Always wear your lifejacket or PFD.
2. Never overload your boat.
3. Step and sit in the middle, boats can tip easily. Never sit on the bow.
4. To operate any boat takes skill. Take lessons.
5. Don't take your boat close to swimmers.
6. Direct the bow of your boat into any big waves.
7. Stay with your boat if it tips over. Swimming to shore can be risky.

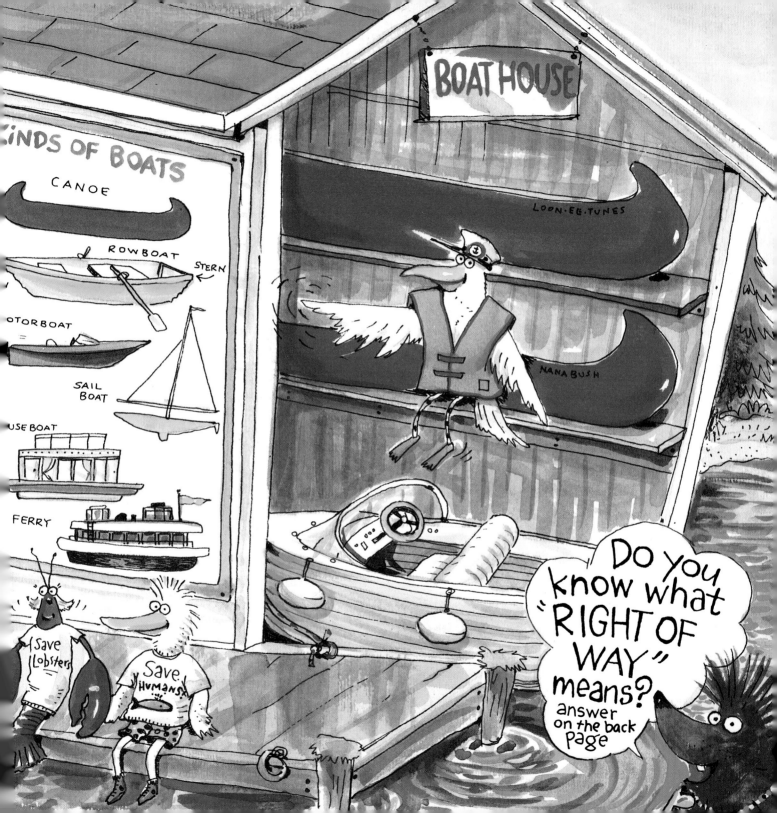

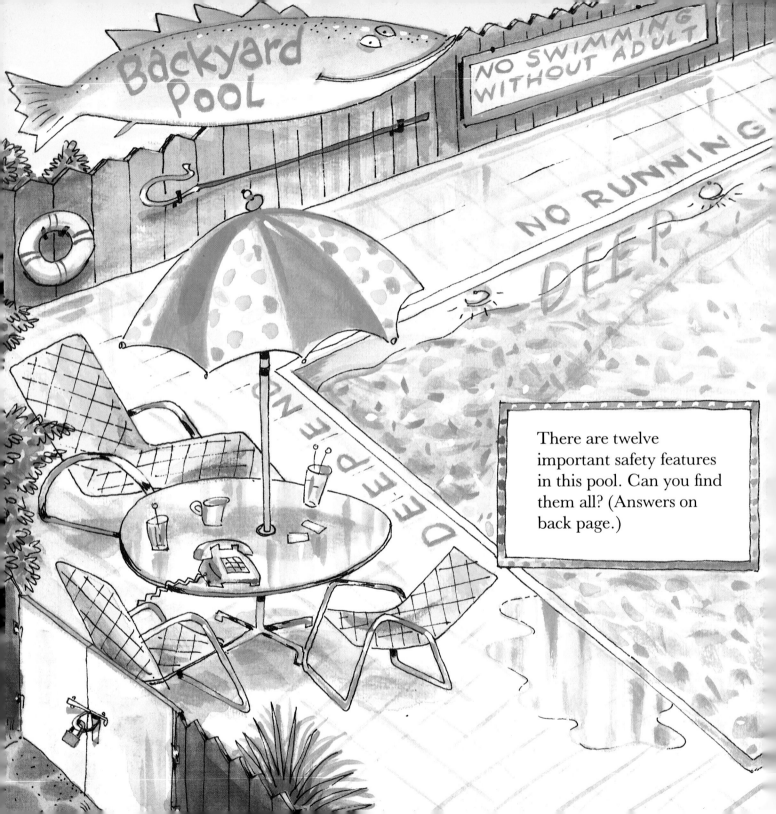

There are twelve important safety features in this pool. Can you find them all? (Answers on back page.)

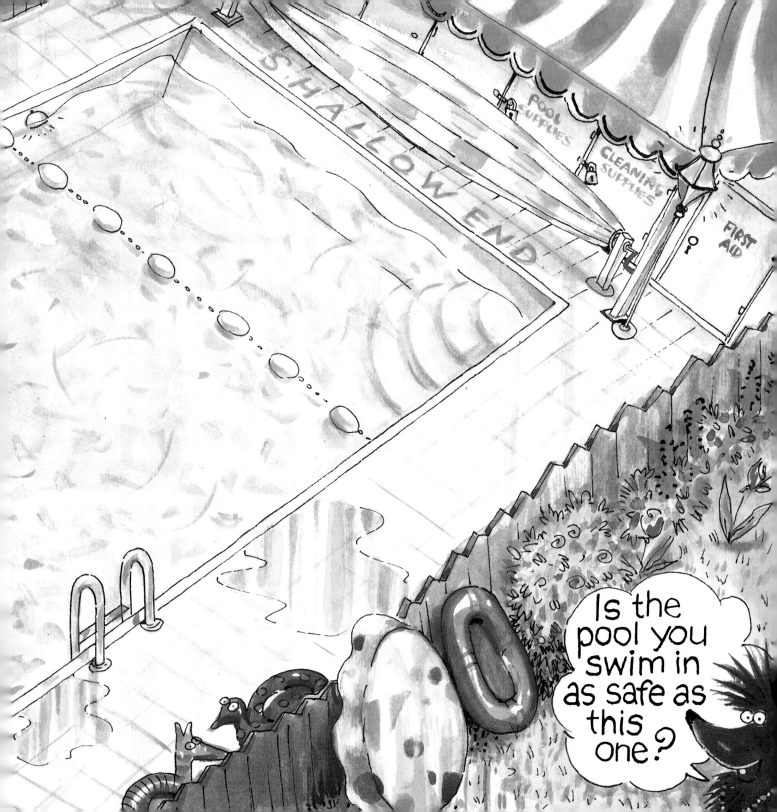

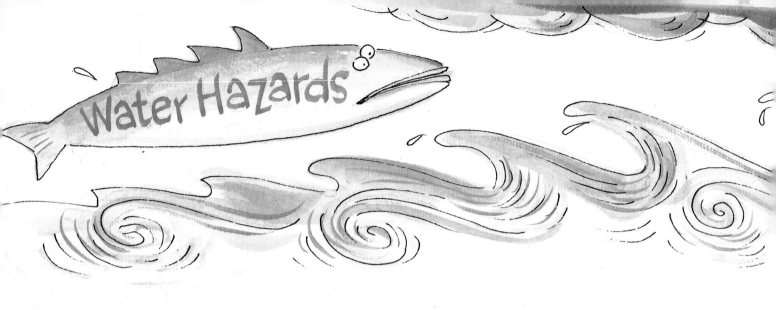

Water Hazards

1. Never jump or dive into unknown, murky, or very cold water.

2. Stay away from fast-moving water in rivers and streams.

3. Remember that rocks and docks can be slippery when wet.

4. Stay away from stagnant water.

5. Water is not always safe for drinking. Check with an adult first.

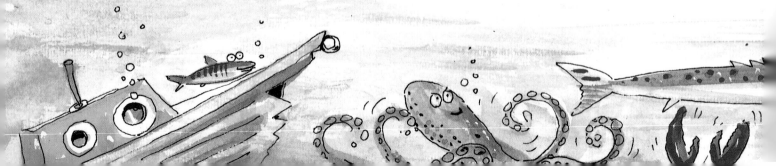

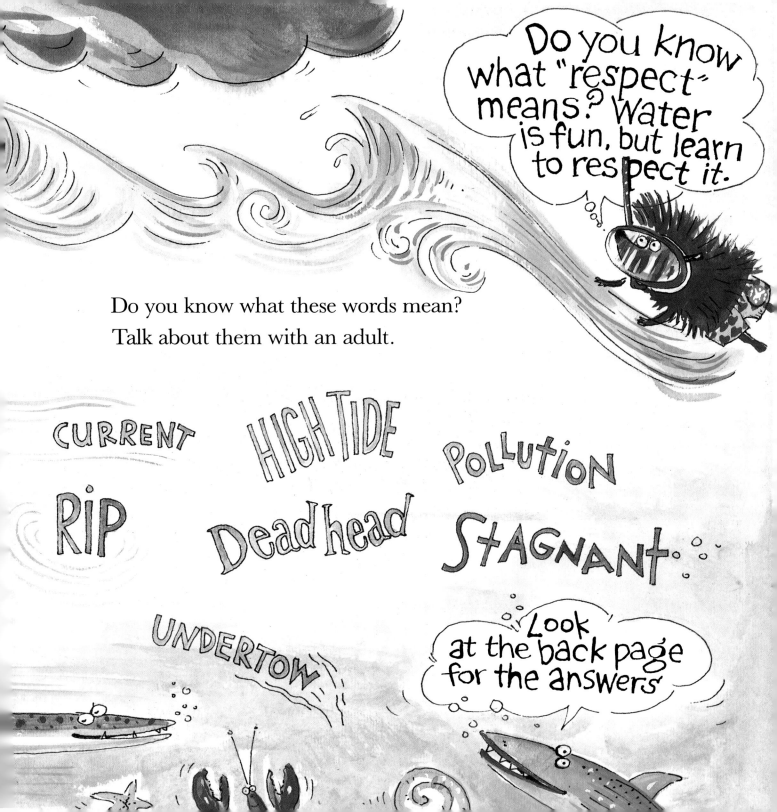

Do you know what "respect" means? Water is fun, but learn to respect it.

Do you know what these words mean?
Talk about them with an adult.

CURRENT

HIGH TIDE

POLLUTION

RIP

Dead head

STAGNANT

UNDERTOW

Look at the back page for the answers

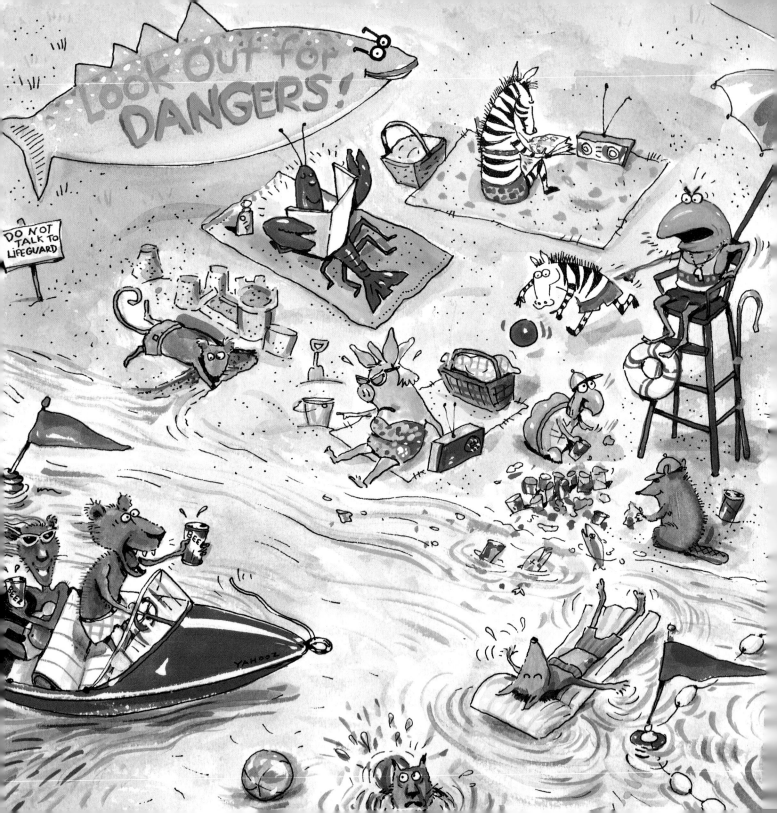

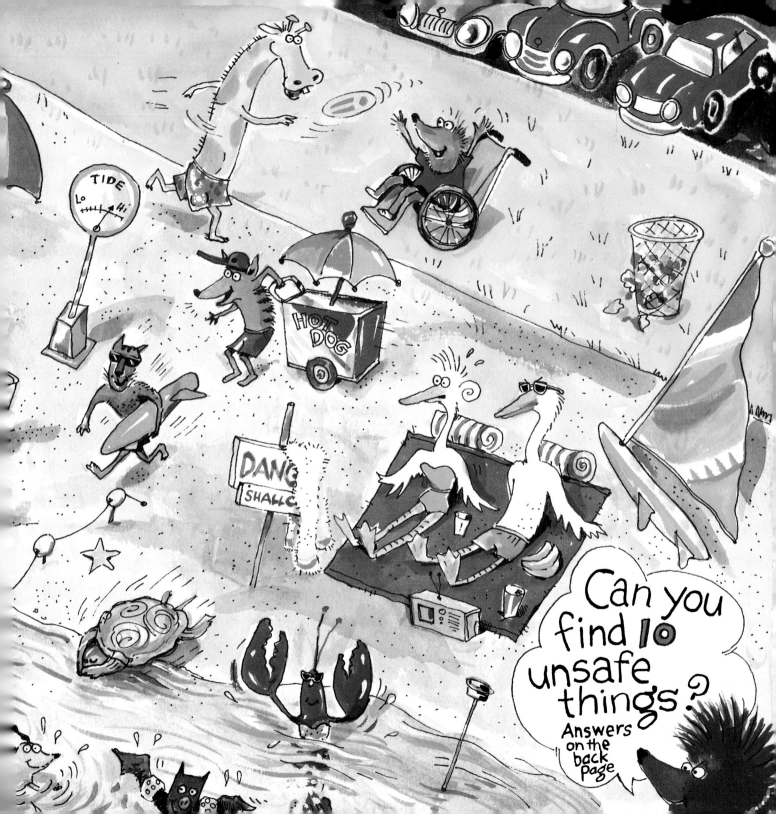

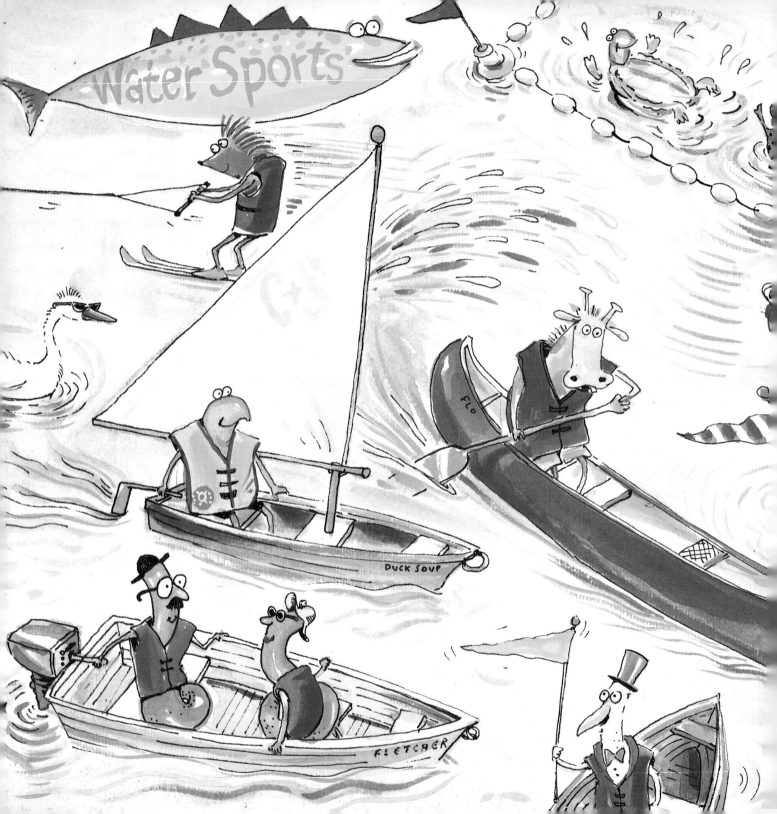

1. Have an adult with you.

2. Learn the correct skills from someone who knows them.

3. Learn the safety rules for each sport.

4. Make sure your equipment works well.

5. Look out for others.

6. Know what to do if you get into difficulty.

Don't waterski or windsurf on a narrow river!

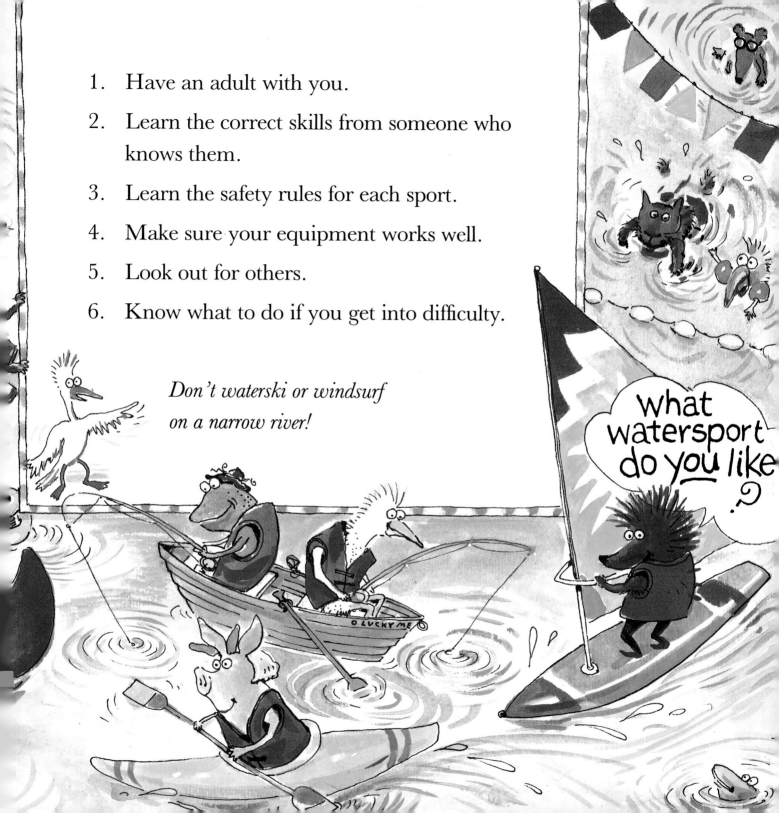

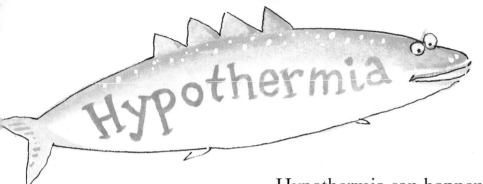 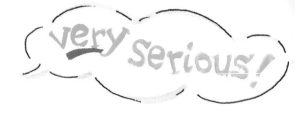

Hypothermia — very serious!

What Is It?

Hypothermia can happen to you if you are in cold water for too long. Your body loses heat and becomes numb. If it loses too much heat, you may become unconscious and unable to help yourself.

What to Look For

Cold, shivering, numbness, drowsiness, bluish skin.

How to Avoid It

NEVER stay in the water when you are chilled or cold.

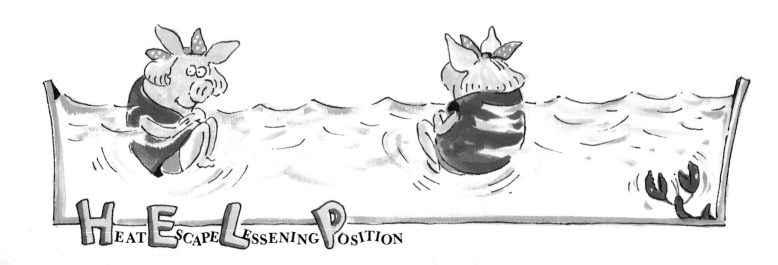

HEAT ESCAPE LESSENING POSITION

What to Do in the Water

1. If your boat tips over, stay with your boat. Try to get as much of your body out of the water as possible. Your body will lose heat quickly in cold water.
2. Keep your clothes on to help you stay warm, but if you are wearing boots, take them off.
3. Stay calm and keep as still as possible.
4. Learn the H.E.L.P. survival position. Hug yourself and tuck your knees up toward your chin.

What to Do When You Get Out

1. Take off all your wet clothing, if you have something dry to put on.
2. Keep warm.
3. Drink something warm.
4. Huddle under a blanket to bring back body heat.
5. Tell an adult.

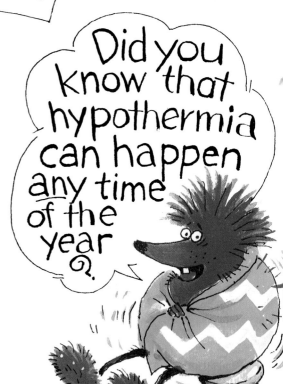

Did you know that hypothermia can happen any time of the year?

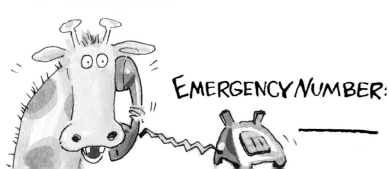

EMERGENCY NUMBER: _____

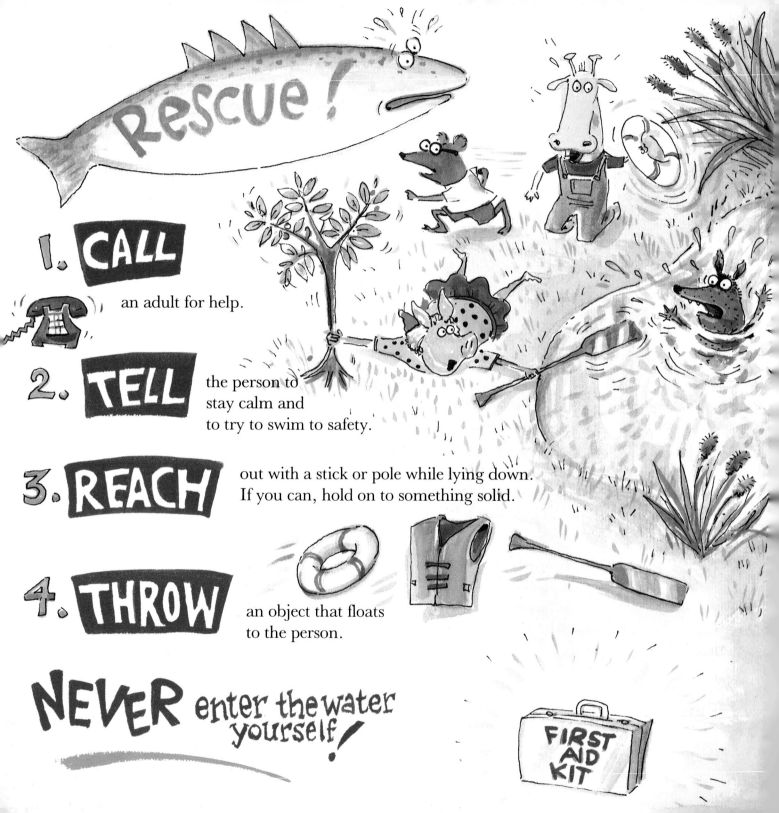

Rescue!

1. **CALL** an adult for help.

2. **TELL** the person to stay calm and to try to swim to safety.

3. **REACH** out with a stick or pole while lying down. If you can, hold on to something solid.

4. **THROW** an object that floats to the person.

NEVER enter the water yourself!

FIRST AID KIT

ice Safety

If You fall through the ICE

1. Don't panic.
2. Call an adult.
3. Spread your arms across the surface of the ice.
4. Kick into a swimming position and slide on to the ice. If the ice breaks, push your way to thicker ice. Roll away from the hole and crawl to safety.

If Someone Else falls through the ICE

1. Call an adult.
2. NEVER go on weakened ice yourself.
3. Try to reach the person with a pole, rope, or stick and pull the person to safety. If you can, hold on to something solid while you reach out.

Do you and your family practise rescue drills?

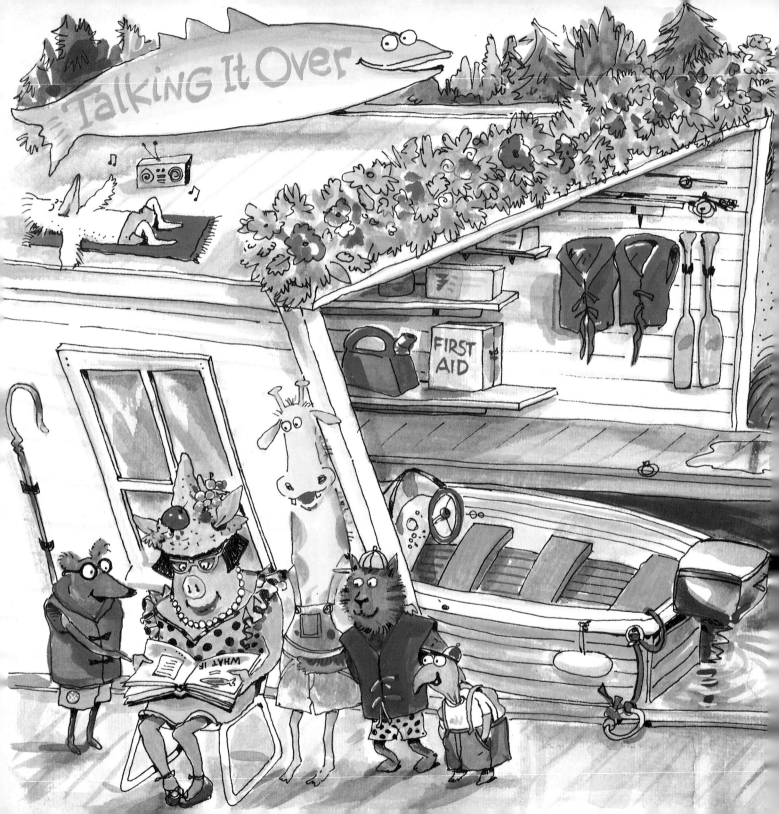

What Would You Do If.......

- Your pet fell into the water?
- There aren't enough lifejackets to go around?
- You are in a boat and you see lightning?
- A dead fish washed ashore?
- There is no lifeguard at the pool?
- You are caught in a current?
- You see a sailboat tip over in a storm?
- You are at a new beach for the first time?

Can you and your parents think of other "What Ifs"?

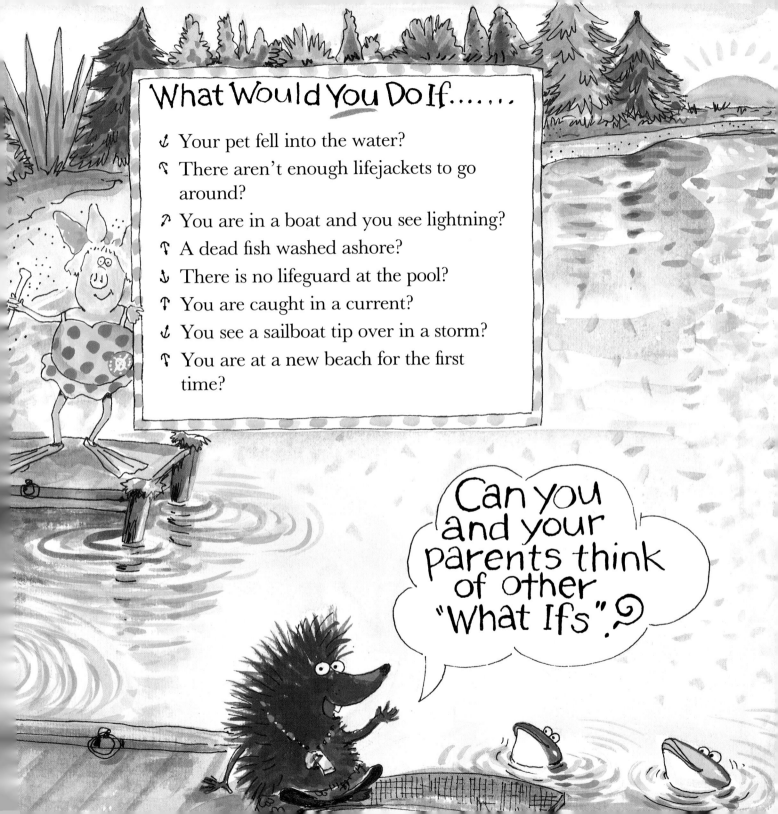

Definitions

Right of way   the right to go first (for example, swimmers have right of way over boaters; sailboats, rowboats, and canoes have right of way over power boats)

Current   a steady movement of running water in one direction

Undertow   the pull of water out to sea following the break-up of a wave on the beach

Rip (Riptide)   fast-flowing currents which are very dangerous

High Tide   the times at the seaside or the ocean when the water reaches its highest level on the beach

Deadhead   a water-soaked log floating at or below the surface of a river or lake

Pollution   the dirtying of water, soil, or air with man-made waste

Stagnant   dull, sluggish water that does not move and has no current; it is usually polluted

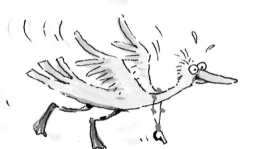

The Badge

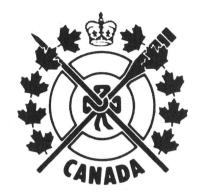

The Royal Life Saving Society Canada offers a sequence of award programs which prepare swimmers to be lifesavers — of themselves and of others. Lifesavers can go on through the Royal Life Saving program to become swimming and lifesaving instructors or lifeguards.

Some of the characters in this book are wearing the Royal Life badge on their bathing suits. Can you find them?

Answers

Look Out for Dangers
1. power boat too close to swimmers and to shore
2. turtle diving into too-shallow water
3. someone swimming outside a designated swim area and chasing a ball out to sea
4. use of air mattress outside of designated swim area: danger of being swept out to sea
5. mother not watching child
6. children playing too close to garbage, rusted cans, broken glass, and dead fish
7. towel hanging over danger sign
8. lobster burning in the sun
9. boaters drinking alcohol
10. boaters not wearing lifejackets

At the Pool
1. ringbuoy
2. high fence around pool
3. locked gate
4. wading pool empty and up against wall
5. first aid supplies
6. cleaning supplies locked in cupboard
7. deep and shallow ends clearly marked
8. safety rules posted
9. telephone
10. buoys dividing deep and shallow ends
11. reaching pole
12. night lights